Intermittent Fasting for Women Over 60: A Guide to Achieve Optimal Health and Longevity

By Dr. Lucille Harris

Table of Contents

Introduction

Our bodies experience significant changes as we age, which may impact our general health and happiness. In addition to reducing cognitive function and physical capacities, these changes can frequently be associated with an increased risk of chronic diseases like heart disease, diabetes, and cancer in women over 60. However, mounting data suggest intermittent fasting may be an effective strategy for enhancing longevity and good health in women over 60.

What is intermittent fasting?

Alternating between times of fasting and eating is referred to as intermittent fasting. Although the practice has been practiced for religious and cultural purposes for millennia, it has become more well-known recently due to its possible health advantages. Numerous health indicators, including insulin sensitivity, blood pressure, cholesterol levels, and inflammation, have been demonstrated in studies to be improved by intermittent fasting. Additionally, it has been demonstrated that intermittent fasting encourages fat and weight loss, which can help lower the chance of developing chronic diseases.

Many women over 60 may be reluctant to start intermittent fasting due to worries about its effectiveness and safety, despite the mounting evidence for its health benefits. Intermittent fasting, however, has the potential to be a secure and reliable method for women over 60 to enhance their health and well-being.

We will examine the facts supporting intermittent fasting for women over 60 in this book and the possible measures you may take to incorporate the practice into your daily routine. This book will provide the methods and skills you need to succeed, whether you are new to intermittent fasting or have tried it previously.

We'll start by learning about the various forms of intermittent fasting and how they affect the body. The advantages of intermittent fasting for women over 60, including its effect on aging and longevity, will be covered in detail. We will next explain how to prepare for and carry out intermittent fasting, along with advice on controlling hunger and cravings.

Next, we'll talk about how crucial it is to balance intermittent fasting and a nutritious diet, providing advice on creating a balanced diet and taking care of your supplements. We will also discuss typical difficulties that may occur during intermittent fasting and methods for resolving them.

We'll finish talking about how crucial it is to keep up intermittent fasting for long-term health and well-being. We'll provide pointers on how to check your progress, add physical exercise to your fasting plan as needed, and change it as necessary.

Benefits of Intermittent fasting

A dietary strategy known as intermittent fasting (IF) involves alternating between periods of eating and fasting. IF has several potential advantages for both physical and mental health. The advantages of intermittent fasting include the following:

1. Weight loss: This is one of the main advantages of intermittent fasting. You eat less overall if you restrict the hours you can eat. The body's metabolism has also been boosted by fasting, making it easier to burn more calories even when at rest.

2. Increased insulin sensitivity: People with obesity, prediabetes, and type 2 diabetes frequently experience insulin resistance, a health risk. By enhancing insulin sensitivity, intermittent fasting can lower the chance of developing diabetes and simplify the body's control of blood sugar levels.

3. Reduced inflammation: Heart disease, cancer, and Alzheimer's disease are just a few health issues linked to chronic inflammation. It has been demonstrated that intermittent fasting reduces inflammation on the body.

4. Improved heart health: By lowering blood pressure, triglyceride, and cholesterol levels, intermittent fasting can help improve heart health.

5. Prolonged lifespan: Mounting data suggests cellular health can be improved, and intermittent fasting can reduce oxidative stress.

6. Better brain health: Studies have indicated that intermittent fasting lowers the risk of neurodegenerative disorders like Alzheimer's and Parkinson's while enhancing cognition, memory, and focus.

7. Reduced risk of cancer: it helps reduce cancer risks such as breast and colon cancer and has been linked to intermittent fasting.

8. Improved gut health: By encouraging the growth of beneficial gut bacteria and lowering digestive tract inflammation, intermittent fasting can enhance gut health.

9. Increased autophagy: The body uses autophagy to eliminate damaged cells and recycle their parts. It has been demonstrated that intermittent fasting increases autophagy, enhancing cellular health and lowering the risk of chronic illnesses.

There are numerous potential advantages of intermittent fasting for physical and mental health. Remembering that these advantages can change based on the person and the precise fasting plan used is crucial. A healthcare practitioner should be consulted before beginning an intermittent fasting plan.

Chapter One
Understanding Intermittent Fasting

A dietary strategy known as intermittent fasting (IF) involves alternating between periods of eating and fasting. Intermittent fasting comes in a variety of forms, each with a unique strategy and advantages. Below are don't of the popular forms of intermittent fasting:

1. Time-restricted feeding: This entails setting a daily time limit on when you can eat. For instance, you might only consume food for 8 hours (say, from midday to 8 p.m.) and observe a 16-hour fast. One of the most well-liked forms of intermittent fasting is this one.

2. Alternate-day fasting: This strategy entails eating normally one day, then fasting the following day. During fasting days, you may only drink water, tea, or other calorie-free beverages.

3. 5:2 Diet plan: Calls for regularly eating five days a week and limiting calories to 500–600 for two days. Another common form of intermittent fasting is this one.

4. Eat-stop-eat: Eat-stop-eat entails going without food for one or two days a week. For instance, you might fast between supper one day and dinner the following.

5. The warrior diet: This strategy entails having one substantial meal at night and going without food during the day. The premise behind this strategy is that this is how our forefathers used to eat.

These many forms of intermittent fasting each have advantages and disadvantages of their own. For instance, time-restricted feeding is straightforward and may aid blood sugar control and weight loss. Although it may be more challenging to maintain, alternate-day fasting can cause significant weight loss and lower the chance of developing chronic diseases. Since the 5:2 diet still permits five days of regular eating each week, it might be more enduring for certain people.

It's crucial to understand that intermittent fasting is not a universal strategy. Finding a sustainable plan that fits your lifestyle and advances your goals is vital because what works for one person may not work for another. Before beginning an intermittent fasting program, speaking with a healthcare provider is advisable, especially if you have a history of disordered eating or other health issues.

How it works in the body

When you fast, your body undergoes changes that can improve your health in several ways.

The body uses glucose and glycogen, stored as energy during fasting periods. When these reserves are depleted, the body metabolizes fat reserves for energy. The result of this process, known as ketosis, is ketone bodies, which the brain and other organs can use as fuel.

Growth hormone levels rise, and insulin levels fall as the body is fasting. This may improve insulin sensitivity, increase fat burning, and increase muscle growth, among other beneficial benefits on health.

It has also been demonstrated that intermittent fasting increases autophagy, a cellular process in which damaged or old cells are decomposed and recycled. This procedure can lower the chance of developing chronic diseases and enhance cellular health.

By encouraging the development of good gut bacteria and lowering digestive tract inflammation, intermittent fasting may also benefit the gut microbiome.

Intermittent fasting can cause behavioral and psychological changes in addition to these physiological ones. For instance, it can aid in lowering snacking and mindless eating, enhancing mindfulness regarding food, and enhancing the body's reaction to hunger signals.

A cleaner gut flora, higher insulin sensitivity, increased fat burning, and improved cellular health are just a few of the advantages of intermittent fasting for the body. It's crucial to remember that depending on the person and the precise fasting plan followed, the consequences of intermittent fasting may differ. Consult with your healthcare practitioner before starting an intermittent fasting plan.

Who can benefit from intermittent fasting

Many people can benefit from intermittent fasting (IF), but it's crucial to remember that not everyone should fast. The following categories of persons may gain from intermittent fasting:

1. Healthy adults: Intermittent fasting may benefit healthy individuals who want to enhance their health and well-being. The benefits of IF are weight loss, better blood sugar regulation, and cardiovascular health.

2. Type 2 diabetics: Because intermittent fasting can increase insulin sensitivity and blood sugar control, it can benefit those with type 2 diabetes.

3. Individuals with Metabolic syndrome: Metabolic syndrome is a group of disorders that includes high blood pressure, excessive blood sugar, extra body fat around the waist, and abnormal cholesterol or triglyceride levels. Some of these issues and the risk of developing chronic diseases with IF may be improved.

4. Women over 60: Intermittent fasting may benefit women over 60 as it can enhance general health and lower the risk of chronic illnesses, including cancer and cardiovascular disease.

Intermittent fasting may benefit some athletes since it can increase fat burning and boost endurance. It's crucial to remember that athletes have unique nutritional requirements, and they should consult a healthcare provider to ensure they meet those requirements while engaging in intermittent fasting.

It's crucial to remember that intermittent fasting is not advised for some people, such as those who are pregnant or nursing, have a history of disordered eating, and have certain medical conditions. Before beginning an intermittent fasting program, speaking with a healthcare provider is crucial, especially if you have a history of medical issues or are currently on medication.

Chapter Two
The Science of Intermittent Fasting for Women Over 60

A dietary strategy known as intermittent fasting (IF) involves alternating between periods of eating and fasting. Fewer research has particularly examined how IF affects women over the age of 60, although many studies have examined the impact of IF on overall health. However, according to the currently available research, IF may offer various advantages to women in this age group.

Improving metabolic health is one of the key advantages of IF for women over 60. Our bodies ability to metabolize glucose declines with age, increasing the risk of type 2 diabetes and other metabolic diseases. IF has been demonstrated to enhance blood sugar regulation and insulin sensitivity, which may assist in lowering the chance of developing these disorders.

Additionally, IF can enhance older women's cardiovascular health. According to studies, IF can lessen inflammatory markers like blood pressure and lipid profiles and lower inflammation, risk factors for cardiovascular disease.

For women over 60, better cognitive function is another advantage of IF. According to studies, IF can raise brain-derived neurotrophic factor (BDNF) levels, a protein essential for brain tissue development and upkeep. Memory, learning, and general cognitive function can all be enhanced by this.

IF lowers the risk of developing some cancers. According to studies, IGF-1 (insulin-like growth factor-1), a hormone associated with an elevated risk of breast and colon cancer, can be decreased by IF.

It's crucial to remember that IF's effects can change according to the precise fasting plan utilized and personal characteristics like age, sex, and general health. Before beginning an IF program, speaking with a healthcare provider is advisable, especially if you have a history of medical issues or are already on medication.

Overall, the evidence indicates that IF may benefit older women in several ways, including better metabolic and cardiovascular health, greater cognitive function, and a decreased risk of some cancers. Even while further studies are required to understand how IF affects this demographic, these results imply that IF might be a useful dietary strategy for older women who want to enhance their general health and well-being.

How aging affects the body

Every aspect of the body is impacted by aging, which is a normal process. Our health and well-being can be impacted by the numerous changes our bodies undergo as we age. Here are a few ways that growing older has an impact on the body:

1. **Loss of muscle mass:** We lose muscle mass as we age, affecting our strength and mobility. Daily tasks may become more challenging, and the danger of falls and accidents may rise.

2. **Reduced bone density:** Age-related bone loss can raise the risk of fractures and osteoporosis. Aging can also cause a decline in bone density.

3. **Reduced metabolism:** As we age, our metabolism tends to slow down, making it harder to keep a healthy weight and raising the risk of diseases like type 2 diabetes.

4. **Atherosclerosis:** (hardening of the arteries), high blood pressure, and other cardiovascular disorders are at higher risk due to aging, which can also cause changes in the cardiovascular system.

5. **Age-related decline in cognitive function:** Aging can also affect memory, attention, and processing speed. This may make daily tasks more challenging and raise the risk of illnesses like dementia and Alzheimer's disease.

6. **Vision and hearing changes:** As we age, our vision and hearing may also deteriorate, affecting our capacity for

communication and awareness of our surroundings.

While these changes are a normal part of aging, there are things we can do to lessen their effects and keep our health and well-being as we become older. This could entail keeping socially active, eating well, getting enough sleep, exercising regularly, and maintaining health as we age can also depend on working with healthcare specialists to handle any underlying medical concerns and staying current on preventive measures.

The impact of intermittent fasting on aging

Recent study indicates intermittent fasting (IF) may also have anti-aging properties. IF has been found to have several advantages for general health and well-being. IF may affect the aging process in several ways, including the following:

1. **An improvement in metabolic health:** As we age, our bodies become less effective at processing glucose, which can raise the risk of type 2 diabetes and other metabolic diseases. It has been demonstrated that IF increases insulin sensitivity and blood sugar regulation, which can lower the chance of developing these illnesses.

2. **Reduced inflammation:** Cancer, Alzheimer's, and cardiovascular disease are only a few age-related illnesses mostly attributed to chronic inflammation. It has been demonstrated that IF lowers inflammatory markers in the body, potentially lowering the risk of several illnesses.

3. IF has been proven to promote autophagy, a process by which the body disassembles and eliminates damaged cells and cellular components, increasing the rate of cellular repair, which will have an anti-aging impact in addition to helping cells perform better.

4. IF has been proven to raise levels of brain-derived neurotrophic factor (BDNF), a protein essential for the development and upkeep of brain cells, which can enhance learning, memory, and general cognitive function.

5. **Protection from aging-related illnesses:** IF may help lower the risk of aging-related illnesses such as cancer, cardiovascular disease, and Alzheimer's disease. Its effects on cellular repair, inflammation, and metabolic health may cause this.

It's crucial to note that additional research is required to completely comprehend the processes by which IF influences the aging process and that the effects of IF on aging are still being explored. A healthcare expert should also be consulted before beginning an IF program, particularly if you have a history of medical issues or are already on medication.

Overall, the research indicates that IF may slow the aging process by enhancing metabolic health, decreasing inflammation, boosting cellular repair, enhancing cognitive function, and defending against age-related disorders. Age-related improvements in general health and well-being may be possible for older persons who include IF in a healthy lifestyle.

Benefits of intermittent fasting for women over 60

It has been revealed that intermittent fasting (IF) has several advantages for general health and well-being, and these advantages may be especially significant for women over 60. The following are some ways that IF could help women in this age group:

Better metabolic health: As women age, their metabolisms may shift, making it harder to maintain a healthy weight and lower the risk of diseases like type 2 diabetes. IF has been demonstrated to enhance blood sugar regulation and insulin sensitivity, which may assist in lowering the chance of developing these disorders.

Reduced inflammation: Chronic inflammation is a major contributor to many age-related illnesses, such as cancer,

Alzheimer's, and cardiovascular disease. IF has been demonstrated to lower inflammatory markers in the body, which may aid in lowering the chance of developing certain illnesses.

Protection from age-related illnesses: IF may help lower the risk of age-related illnesses like cancer, Alzheimer's, and cardiovascular disease, which might result from how it affects cellular repair, inflammation, and metabolic health.

Enhancement of cognitive function: Research has indicated that IF raises levels of brain-derived neurotrophic factor (BDNF), a protein essential for developing and upkeep brain cells. Memory, learning, and general cognitive function can all be enhanced by this.

Increased longevity: IF has been found to lengthen life in experiments on animals, and some evidence points to potential human applications for this effect. IF may support longevity by lowering the risk of age-related illnesses and enhancing general health.

It's crucial to remember that IF's effects on women over 60 are still being researched, and more studies are required to comprehend this dietary strategy's potential advantages and risks properly. Before beginning an IF program, speaking with a healthcare provider is advisable, especially if you have a history of medical issues or are already on medication.

Overall, the research indicates that IF may help older women in several ways, including better metabolic health, less inflammation, defense against age-related disorders, improved cognitive function, and increased longevity. Older women can enhance their general health and well-being as they age by including IF in a healthy lifestyle.

The role of autophagy in intermittent fasting

The body uses the cellular process of autophagy to degrade and reuse proteins, organelles, and other cellular components that are damaged or malfunctioning. Maintaining cellular health and function depends on this mechanism, which may also contribute significantly to the advantages of intermittent fasting (IF).

The body utilizes stored fat instead of glucose as its fasting fuel source. An increase in autophagy is one of a series of cellular changes brought on by this switch. The body starts to break down and recycle damaged proteins and other cellular components to produce energy and preserve cellular function.

Many factors make autophagy crucial. In the beginning, it aids in removing harmed or defective organelles and proteins, which might amass over time and obstruct cellular function. Autophagy assists in maintaining healthy, effective cells by recycling these parts.

Second, autophagy is crucial for cellular regeneration and repair. The body can produce new, healthy components to replace damaged ones by disassembling and recycling the broken ones.

Finally, autophagy might slow down the aging process. Age-related disorders and decline can be exacerbated by the body's decreased ability to remove harmed proteins and other cellular components as we age. IF may aid in slowing this process and promoting healthy aging by boosting autophagy.

Even while the benefits of autophagy in IF are still being researched, new evidence points to this cellular activity as a potential cornerstone to this dietary strategy's anti-aging and health-improving impacts. IF may contribute to cellular health improvement, inflammation reduction, and general health and well-being by inducing autophagy.

Chapter Three
Preparing for Intermittent Fasting

It's critical to emotionally and physically prepare for intermittent fasting if you want to succeed with it. Here are some pointers to get you going:

Before beginning an intermittent fasting schedule, learn about the various fasting methods and their potential advantages and disadvantages. The 16/8 method, in which you fast for 16 hours and eat within an 8-hour window, and the 5:2 approach, in which you usually eat for five days and limit your calorie intake to 500–600 calories on two separate days, are two examples of popular fasting schedules.

1. **Start slowly:** It's best to ease into intermittent fasting if you're a beginner. Start with shorter fasts, perhaps 12

hours, and progressively extend them as your body gets used to them.

2. **Meal planning:** Maintaining your fasting schedule and resisting temptation is essential. To feed your body throughout your non-fasting periods, incorporate wholesome, nutrient-dense foods in your meals.

3. **Keep hydrated:** Water helps to keep you hydrated and reduces appetite, so drinking plenty of it when fasting is essential. Aim to consume eight glasses of water or more each day.

4. **Get enough sleep:** Sleep is crucial during a fast since it controls your metabolism and hunger. To make sure that your body is well-rested and ready to face the day, aim for 7-8 hours of sleep each night.

5. **Regular exercise:** Exercising regularly can enhance your overall health and speed up your metabolism. When fasting, paying attention to your energy levels and modifying your workout plan as necessary is crucial.

6. **Seek assistance:** Intermittent fasting can be challenging, especially at first. To keep motivated and accountable, enlist the aid of friends, family, or a group of people who share your values.

Set yourself up for a successful intermittent fasting journey by following these suggestions. You'll be well on your way to enjoying the many advantages of this well-liked dieting strategy if you keep in mind to be patient with yourself and pay attention to your body's demands.

Understanding your body's needs

Any effective intermittent fasting regimen, especially for women, must consider the body's needs. Cycling between fasting and non-fasting phases is a common dieting strategy known as intermittent fasting. While weight loss and better blood sugar management are only two advantages of intermittent fasting for women, it's critical to recognize your body's particular requirements for success.

When creating an intermittent fasting regimen, women should take the following essential elements into account:

Menstrual cycle: During the menstrual cycle, women's bodies experience hormonal changes that may impact their appetite, level of energy, and general well-being. It's crucial to be aware of these variations and modify your fasting regimen as necessary. For instance, although some women may prefer to fast during the luteal phase (the second half of the cycle) when progesterone levels are more significant, others may find it beneficial to fast during the follicular phase (the first half of the menstrual cycle), when estrogen levels are higher.

1. **Calorie requirements:** Due to differences in body size, composition, hormonal, and metabolic processes, women have different calorie requirements than men. It's crucial to calculate your daily caloric demands depending on your unique characteristics, like your age, height, weight, and level of exercise, and to modify your fasting schedule accordingly.

2. **Nutritional requirements:** Women have particular nutritional requirements throughout particular life periods like

pregnancy and lactation. Consume enough critical nutrients throughout your non-fasting periods, such as iron, calcium, and folic acid, to support your general health.

3. **Energy level:** Women may have varying degrees of energy while intermittent fasting, particularly in the beginning. It's important to pay attention to your body's signs and adjust your fasting schedule as necessary. For instance, you should break your fast early or change your fasting schedule if you feel tired or dizzy.

4. **Psychological factors:** Stress, emotional eating, and body image concerns are just a few examples of the psychological issues that women may have that may make it difficult for them to follow an intermittent fasting

schedule. It's critical to be aware of these circumstances and create coping mechanisms, such as mindfulness exercises and asking friends and family for assistance.

By understanding your body's unique requirements, you can create an intermittent fasting schedule customized to your needs and preferences. You'll be well on your way to enjoying the many advantages of this well-liked dieting strategy if you keep paying attention to your body's cues and modify your fasting schedule as necessary.

Pre-fasting assessment and consultation

Cycling between times of eating and fasting is a common weight loss and health-promoting method known as intermittent fasting (IF). Although IF can be a valuable method for shedding pounds and enhancing health, it is crucial to speak with a healthcare professional before beginning IF, mainly if you are a woman.

Women must speak with a healthcare professional before beginning IF for several reasons:

- Women's nutritional requirements differ from those of men's. For instance, women require more calcium and iron than males do.

- Compared to men, women might be more susceptible to the effects of fasting. Women, for instance, could become more lethargic or experience mood fluctuations during fasting.

- Certain medical conditions, like pregnancy or diabetes, may make IF risky for some women.

A healthcare professional can assist you in deciding if IF is the best option for you as well as in creating a plan that is both secure and efficient. Your healthcare professional will inquire about your medical history, eating and exercise routine, and IF goals during the pre-fasting assessment. They might also conduct blood tests to evaluate your levels of iron, calcium, and other nutrients.

Once you have been given the all-clear for IF, your healthcare practitioner can assist you in creating a strategy that works for you specifically. This strategy may consist of the following:

- A set period of fasting

- A list of the items you should consume throughout your eating window.
- A list of foods to stay away from during the fasting period.
- Guidelines for controlling cravings and hunger.
- Advice on how to remain hydrated.

When beginning IF, it's critical to adhere to your healthcare provider's advice carefully. Stop using IF and consult your doctor if you develop any unfavorable side effects, including exhaustion, mood fluctuations, or dizziness.

For women who are thinking about IF, here are some extra suggestions:

- Begin gradually. Start with a shorter fasting window, like 12 hours, if you are new to intermittent fasting. As you become more accustomed to IF, gradually lengthen your fasting window.

- Be aware of your body. Break your fast if you feel worn out, dizzy, or ill.

- Remain hydrated. Consume plenty of water, unsweetened tea, and coffee throughout your fasting window.

- Adopt a balanced diet. During your dining window, be sure to consume a lot of fruits, veggies, and whole grains.

- Exercise regularly. You can burn calories and enhance your general health by exercising.

- Speak with your healthcare professional. Before beginning IF, discuss any health issues with your healthcare physician.

- It is crucial to speak with a healthcare professional if you are a woman thinking about IF to ensure it is safe. IF can be a secure and reliable strategy to reduce weight and enhance your health with the proper preparation and direction.

How to choose the right fasting plan

The optimal intermittent fasting (IF) plan for you will depend on your particular requirements and objectives. There are numerous IF plans available. When selecting an IF plan, keep the following things in mind:

Your lifestyle: Different IF programs offer different levels of flexibility. If you have a busy life, select a plan like the 16:8 diet that allows you to eat at specific times of the day.

Your Health: Before beginning IF, you should discuss any medical issues you may have, like diabetes or pregnancy, with your doctor. People with specific medical issues may not be able to use some IF schemes safely.

Your targets: Choose a diet restricting your calorie consumption during fasting if weight loss is your primary goal. Choose a plan that emphasizes eating healthy foods within your eating window to enhance your general health.

After taking them into account, you can begin researching other IF plans.

Tips for managing hunger and cravings

Here are some pointers for controlling hunger and cravings while fasting intermittently:

Stay Hydrated: Drink a lot of water to stay hydrated and stave off hungry sensations.

Coffee, unsweetened tea, and water are all sensible options.

Maintain a balanced diet throughout your eating window: Consuming many fruits, veggies, and whole grains might help you stay satisfied and full.

Get enough sleep: When well-rested, you're less likely to experience hunger and cravings.
Avoid sugary beverages: Drinks with added sugar might raise blood sugar levels and cause cravings later.

Discover healthy diversion strategies: If you start to feel hungry or in need, attempt to divert your attention with something else, such as reading, taking a walk, or listening to music.
Feel free to break your fast if you're feeling hungry or ill. Breaking your fast is preferable to pushing yourself too much and being ill.

It's also critical to remember that hunger and cravings are common during intermittent fasting. The goal is to handle them healthily. You may successfully control your hunger and desires with some work, helping you lose weight.

Here are some more ideas that could be useful:

- Planning your meals and snacks will prevent you from making poor decisions when you're anxious or hungry.
- Have a supply of wholesome snacks on hand, so you have something to eat in case of hunger.
- You'll feel fuller after you eat if you take time and taste your food.
- If you feel full, stop eating. Pay attention to your body. You don't have to clear your plate.
- Exercise frequently: Hunger and desires can be reduced with exercise.

- Get enough sleep: When well-rested, you're less likely to experience hunger and cravings.
- Control your stress: Stress can increase appetite and cravings. Find strategies for stress reduction such as meditation, yoga, or physical activity.

You can master controlling hunger and cravings and use intermittent fasting to lose weight with some work successfully.

Chapter Four
Nutrition basics for women over 60

It's crucial to prioritize nutrient-dense foods and satisfy particular nutritional needs regarding nutrition fundamentals for women over 60 who practice intermittent fasting (IF). Below are some important tips to remember:

- **Adequate protein intake:** Our bodies need more protein as we age to promote muscle health and prevent age-related muscle loss. To meet your protein requirements throughout eating times, incorporate protein-rich foods like lean meats, poultry, fish, eggs, dairy products, legumes, and plant-based protein sources like tofu and tempeh.

- **Calcium and vitamin D:** These are essential for maintaining bone health and preventing osteoporosis in women over 60. Include foods high in calcium, such as dairy products, fortified plant-based milk, leafy greens, and tofu that have been calcium-set. Ensure appropriate vitamin D consumption by consuming fatty fish, egg yolks, fortified meals, or getting enough sun exposure.

- **Foods high in fiber:** Eating a diet high in fiber can help you lose weight, control your weight, and lower your chance of developing chronic diseases. To achieve your fiber requirements, eat plenty of fruits, vegetables, whole grains, legumes, nuts, and seeds. Additionally, these foods supply vital vitamins and minerals.

- **Heart-healthy fats:** choose healthy fats that also satisfy you over unhealthy fats. Include olive oil, almonds, seeds, avocados, and fatty fish like mackerel and salmon. Additionally, these fats help the body absorb fat-soluble vitamins.

- **Hydration:** Staying hydrated throughout mealtimes is crucial because older persons may have diminished thirst sense. Consider including herbal teas, infused water, or other hydrating drinks without sugar in addition to your regular water intake.

- **Meals rich in Micronutrients:** Include a variety of vibrant fruits and vegetables in your diet to ensure you're getting a mix of vitamins, minerals, and antioxidants. These vitamins and minerals promote general health and aid in preventing age-related illnesses.

- **Supplements, if required:** Supplementation may be advised based on a person's needs and specific nutritional deficits. To ascertain whether any supplements, such as vitamin B12, omega-3 fatty acids, or multivitamins, are required for you, speak with a healthcare provider or registered dietitian.

- **Eating mindfully:** Make an effort to eat mindfully whenever you have a meal. Watch for signs of hunger and fullness, eat gently, and enjoy your food. You can avoid overeating and make better dietary decisions due to this.

Remember, if you have any specific dietary issues or medical illnesses or are on medication, you should speak with a healthcare provider or trained dietitian to ensure your nutritional needs are addressed while engaging in intermittent fasting. They can help you maximize your nutrition while doing IF by offering individualized advice based on your needs.

Foods to eat and avoid during intermittent fasting

Even though the timing of your meals is limited during intermittent fasting (IF), it's still critical to concentrate on consuming nutrient-dense foods that promote your general health and well-being. To maintain an intermittent fast, the following foods should be consumed and avoided:

Foods to Eat:

Lean protein: Such as poultry, fish, lean meat cuts, eggs, lentils, and tofu. Protein encourages satiety and assists in maintaining muscular mass.

Whole grains: Choose whole grains like quinoa, brown rice, whole wheat bread, and oats from the list below. They deliver minerals, vitamins, fiber, and long-lasting energy.

Veggies and fruits: Add a range of vibrantly colored fruits and veggies to your meals. They are filled with fiber antioxidants, minerals as well as vitamins.

Healthy fats: during Intermittent fasting, choose healthy fats such as those found in avocados, nuts, seeds, olive oil, and fatty seafood. These fats help keep the heart healthy and make you feel full.

Dairy or dairy alternatives: For calcium and protein, if tolerated, consume dairy products or their substitutes, such as yogurt, cheese, or fortified plant-based milk.

Water, herbal teas, and calorie-free beverages can help you stay hydrated while fasting and eating.

Avoid these foods:

Foods high in added sugars, such as sugary drinks, candy, pastries, and processed snacks, should be limited or avoided. These foods can cause energy slumps and help people gain weight.

White bread, white rice, and processed cereals are refined grains that should be avoided. These could produce sharp drops in blood sugar levels because of their higher glycemic index.

Avoid eating foods high in calories and fat, such as fast food, fried foods, and high-fat snacks. They may make it more challenging to lose weight and have a detrimental effect on general health.

Beverages with added sugar: Avoid sugary beverages, including soda, juices with added sugar, energy drinks, and flavored coffees. They include a lot of added sugar and are high in empty calories.

Alcohol abuse: Keep your alcohol intake to a minimum, as it might harm your health and make it challenging to achieve your fasting goals.

This advice is meant to be broad so paying attention to your body and making changes per your unique requirements and dietary preferences is crucial. Additionally, if you have particular nutritional issues or medical conditions, you should get specialized guidance from a healthcare provider or certified dietitian.

Strategies for healthy meal planning

A healthy and balanced diet during intermittent fasting (IF) depends on effective meal planning. Here are some tips to assist you in creating wholesome meals that suit your fasting objectives:

When choosing your meals, prioritize foods high in vital nutrients, such as fruits, vegetables, whole grains, lean meats, and healthy fats. A variety of vitamins, minerals, and antioxidants are included in these foods, supporting general health.

1. Include a range of macronutrients: A mix of carbohydrates, proteins, and fats should be present at each meal. Energy comes from carbohydrates, while proteins and lipids help you feel full and support your body's operations. Including various macronutrients

in your diet can keep you full and well-fed during fasting and eating times.

2. Putting fiber first Fruits, vegetables, whole grains, legumes, and nuts are fiber-rich diets that can improve overall gut health by promoting satiety and regulating digestion. To ensure you're reaching your daily fiber requirements, incorporate a variety of fiber sources into your meals.

3. Focus on staying hydrated: sip on water frequently throughout the day, both when fasting and when eating. Drinking enough water can make you feel fuller between meals and benefit your general health.

4. Make meals that contain a supply of lean protein (for example, poultry, fish, or tofu), complex carbs (for example, whole grains or sweet potatoes), and healthy fats (for example, avocados, nuts, or olive oil). This mixture

assists in giving you long-lasting energy and keeping you full.

5. Batch cooking and meal preparation: This can help you save time and guarantee that you always have nutritious food. Large quantities of grains, veggies, and proteins can be prepared ahead of time and divided into meals. This makes it simpler to assemble balanced meals during your eating times swiftly.

6. Choose smaller, more often meals: Instead of three substantial meals, consider eating smaller, more regular meals or snacks. By doing so, you can control your hunger and avoid overeating.

7. Observe your body:
- Pay attention to your body's signs of fullness and hunger.
- Eat slowly and mindfully, stopping when you are comfortably full.

Always remember that finding a sustainable eating pattern that works for you is the goal of intermittent fasting, not restriction or deprivation.

8. Seek expert advice: If you have particular dietary concerns or medical issues, you should speak with a qualified dietician. They can offer you individualized advice and assist you in developing a food plan that incorporates intermittent fasting and fits your nutritional demands.

Some trial and error may be necessary to find the meal-planning techniques that are most effective for you. Be versatile and flexible, and be bold and try out new recipes and meal combinations. The objective of your intermittent fasting journey is to develop a nourishing and sustainable eating strategy.

Managing supplements and medications during fasting

Thinking about how supplements and drugs could affect your fasting schedule when using intermittent fasting (IF) is crucial. Here are some tips for efficiently managing supplements and medications during IF:

Consult a healthcare practitioner: It's essential to speak with a healthcare provider before beginning IF, especially if you regularly take drugs or have specific medical issues. They can advise you on whether IF is appropriate for you and, if so, how to change your medication plan.

Time your drug intake properly: If your prescription needs to be taken with meals, you should schedule your eating time accordingly. In accordance with the medication schedule, adjust your fasting and eating windows as your healthcare provider recommends.

If you are worried about possible medication interactions and fasting interactions, speak with your pharmacist. They can notify you of any factors to remember during IF or whether specific drugs should be used with food.

Supplements should be taken when eating: Some accessories, particularly those that are fat-soluble or need food for optimal absorption, should be taken with meals. Include supplements that need food or particular nutrients throughout your eating times for better absorption. This guarantees that you get the most out of your nutrients.

Think about water-soluble vitamins: They can be consumed on an empty stomach during fasting time with little to no adverse effects. Examples include vitamin C and the

B-complex vitamins. Without food, these vitamins are typically effectively absorbed, but it's better to adhere to the directions on the supplement container or get advice from a healthcare provider.

Keep yourself hydrated: It's crucial to keep yourself hydrated, even when fasting. Take drugs with a glass of water to facilitate optimal absorption and avoid dehydration.

Herbal supplements should be used cautiously because some may have particular consumption guidelines and interact negatively with medications or fasting objectives. To effectively incorporate herbal supplements during IF, speak with a doctor, nurse, or pharmacist.

Follow your body's reaction: Keep track of how your body reacts to prescription drugs and dietary supplements when fasting and eating.

Consult a medical expert for more advice if you encounter any adverse effects or worries.

Everyone has different needs for supplements and medications, so getting individualized guidance from a doctor or pharmacist is crucial. They can offer personalized advice based on your prescriptions, medical circumstances, and objectives. You can practice intermittent fasting and maintain your health and well-being by properly managing your supplements and medications.

Chapter Five
Overcoming Challenges and Adapting to Intermittent Fasting

As you get used to this eating pattern, intermittent fasting (IF) might present some difficulties. However, with the correct approaches, you can overcome these problems and turn IF into a satisfying and lasting lifestyle choice. Below are some obstacles to overcome:

- **Initial hunger and cravings:** As your body adjusts to the new eating pattern throughout the adjustment period, you can experience increased hunger and desires. To help you feel satiated for longer, stay hydrated, eat fiber-rich meals, and include healthy fats and proteins during your mealtimes. Take part in pursuits that divert your attention from urges, such as taking a stroll or engaging in a pastime.

- **Social circumstances and timing of meals:** Maintaining an intermittent fasting schedule might be difficult during social events or get-togethers that entail food. Adjust your eating or fasting window in advance to account for these occurrences. Share your nutritional choices with loved ones, and emphasize interacting more than just eating. You are also welcome to bring healthy snacks or meals that fit your meal plan.

- **Lack of energy or focus:** During the early phases of IF, energy levels are prone to change. To provide your body with enough fuel during your eating intervals, ensure you're eating meals high in nutrients. To support your energy levels, stay hydrated and prioritize excellent sleep. Your energy levels may stabilize and even increase as your body adapts to the fasting regimen.

- **Digestive Changes:** When beginning intermittent fasting, some people may suffer changes in their bowel motions or digestive pain. Ensure you get enough fiber throughout mealtimes from fruits, veggies, and whole grains. Drink plenty of water to aid in proper digestion. Consult a certified nutritionist or healthcare provider for more advice if your digestive problems don't go away.

- **Plateau or weight loss stalls:** Weight loss can still progress after a plateau or halt, even when using intermittent fasting. To ensure you're in a calorie deficit, assess your calorie intake during mealtimes. Aim for a balance of macronutrients and consider the quality of your meal selections. Strength training and physical activity should be included to aid with weight loss and general health.

- **Emotional and psychological challenges:** Changes in eating patterns may result in emotional and psychological difficulties, such as stress eating or emotional eating. Use stress-reduction strategies like mindfulness meditation or take up a hobby you enjoy. To share your experiences and receive motivation, seek help from friends, family, or a support group.

- **Listening to your body:** Because each person is different, paying attention to your body's indications when engaging in intermittent fasting is essential. Pay attention to your feelings of hunger, satiety, and energy. Find a routine that works best for you by adjusting your fasting and eating windows as necessary. Consult a medical expert if you have any bothersome or persistent symptoms.

It takes time and perseverance to adjust to intermittent fasting. You are choosing a strategy that complements your way of life and promotes your general well-being. Be adaptable, try various fasting patterns, and get help when needed. You may overcome obstacles and successfully implement intermittent fasting if you are persistent and have a good outlook.

Managing stress and self-care during fasting

A healthy lifestyle must prioritize self-care and stress management, mainly during intermittent fasting (IF). Here are some techniques to aid you in practicing self-care and stress management while fasting:

Get adequate sleep: Stress management and general well-being depend on getting enough good sleep. Sleep for 7-9 hours each night, undisturbed. Create a bedtime regimen that encourages relaxation, such as staying away from electronics an hour before bed and fostering a peaceful sleeping atmosphere.

Practice stress-reduction strategies: Take part in stress-reduction methods, including yoga, mindfulness, deep breathing exercises, and meditation. Incorporate what works best for you into your daily routine.

Drink plenty of water: to stay adequately hydrated throughout your fasting and eating intervals. Dehydration can contribute to weariness and higher levels of stress. Always keep a water bottle on you as a reminder to hydrate.

Exercise regularly: Exercise is a great way to reduce stress and can lift your spirits. Make time for activities you enjoy and incorporate them into your daily schedule. This can entail taking a stroll, running, cycling, dancing, or fitness classes. Aim for about 150 minutes or more weekly of moderate-intensity exercise.

Practice mindful eating: To improve your entire experience, practice mindful eating during mealtimes. Take your time, enjoy every bite, and heed your body's hunger and fullness signals. This can facilitate a healthier relationship with food and help minimize eating-related stress.

Take part in fun activities: Schedule time for leisurely pursuits that will help you unwind. This could be hobbies like gardening, reading, listening to music, listening to podcasts, or spending time with loved ones. Spend time doing what makes you happy and relaxes you throughout the day.

Connect with others: Social support is crucial for stress management and preserving a good outlook. To share your experiences, seek support, have meaningful conversations, and contact friends, family, or support groups. Creating and maintaining solid relationships can give one a sense of support and belonging.

Set realistic goals: Having reasonable expectations will help you avoid putting undue pressure on yourself to succeed at intermittent fasting. Accept flexibility and recognize that change takes time. Set attainable objectives and acknowledge your progress along the way. Keep in mind that self-care entails treating oneself nicely and developing self-compassion.

Seek professional assistance: If stress starts to interfere with your everyday life or becomes unbearable, you should talk to a mental health counselor or a member of the medical profession. They can offer direction, tips, and individualized support to help you properly manage your stress.

Whether you engage in intermittent fasting or not, self-care and stress management are crucial components of your well-being. Setting these habits as a top priority can assist you in overcoming the difficulties of IF and leading a healthier, more well-rounded existence.

Conclusion

Congratulations! This fantastic journey through the world of intermittent fasting has ended. You are better prepared than ever to take control of your health and well-being because you are armed with knowledge, valuable strategies, and the drive to change your life.

A method with scientific support, intermittent fasting has transformed how we view food and our bodies. It is not just a fad. You can optimize your metabolism, increase your energy, and even slow aging by using fasting and feasting.

You have investigated the various forms of intermittent fasting throughout this book, learned how it affects your body, and learned how to overcome obstacles and adjust to this life-changing practice. You've discovered the incredible effects of fasting on aging, the mysteries of autophagy, and the unique advantages this effective practice offers women over 60.

But remember that intermittent fasting involves more than when and what you eat. It involves adopting a holistic strategy for your health. It involves feeding your body nutrient-dense foods, engaging in self-care activities, controlling stress levels, and developing a positive outlook.

I urge you to pay attention to your body, respect its needs, and treat yourself kindly as you start this new chapter of your life. Accept the adaptability of intermittent fasting, integrate it into your way of life, and let it inspire you to live life to the fullest.

So, with the information and resources you've gained, proceed confidently. Accept the power of IF and open opportunities for a healthier, happier you. Your path to optimum health starts right now. Prepare yourself to grow, flourish, and realize your full potential.

Remember that intermittent fasting gives you the power to change your life. Accept it, have confidence in yourself, and let the fantastic trip happen. Get ready to unlock your true potential and enjoy the incredible benefits that await you.

Here's to a future brimming with limitless opportunities, a life of vibrant health, and endless energy. We wish you luck on your intermittent fasting journey!